MW01178660

THE PALEO
Pantry

26 Classic Comfort Foods That You Can Stop Buying And Start Making
(Primal Gluten Free Cookbook)

Kate Evans Scott

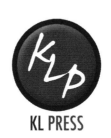

KL PRESS

DISCLAIMER

No part of this publication may be reproduced or transmitted in any form or by any means, mechanical or electronic, including photocopying or recording, or by any information storage and retrieval system, or transmitted by email without permission in writing from the publisher.

Although the author and publisher have made every effort to ensure that the information in this book was correct at press time, the author and publisher do not assume and hereby disclaim any liability to any party for any loss, damage, or disruption caused by errors or omissions, whether such errors or omissions result from negligence, accident, or any other cause.

This book is not intended as a substitute for the medical advice of physicians. The reader should regularly consult a physician in matters relating to his/her health and particularly with respect to any symptoms that may require diagnosis or medical attention.

This book is dedicated to my two beautiful children.

ACKNOWLEDGMENTS

Thank You to my friends and family for your encouragement.
Your support has been the cornerstone of this creative process.

A special thanks also goes out to you the reader ~ I am grateful to
be sharing this journey to health and happiness together with you.

CONTENTS

THE HOMEMADE PALEO PANTRY

I know what you're thinking... You're thinking that if you're Paleo, you're pretty much doing it from scratch. Am I right? Well, I partly agree with you. While we aren't eating all the prepackaged food products that our non-Paleo friends are eating, I'm sure many of us aren't doing it totally from scratch.

Don't get me wrong, I am not knocking you for picking up a carton of organic chicken stock or a bag of frozen vegetables. I don't mind if you buy your pound of grass-fed butter in gold foil wrapping. But my food bill is pretty expensive for my little family, and if anything, doing it from scratch helps me save money... not to mention, everything tastes so much better when it's fresh.

USE EVERYTHING

Do you think our Neanderthal ancestors threw away bits of hard-earned meat? Do you think they tossed out the tips of the celery or discarded the chicken gizzards? I can bet you they did not. Would you throw away one bit of beef if you had to chase the cow down for miles and miles with a spear? Not likely.

My philosophy is to use as much of everything I buy as humanly possible... and compost the rest. For example, a chicken or turkey carcass never goes into the trash. It goes into the slow-cooker to make soup stock. The nut pulp left over from making almond milk doesn't go down the drain, it gets saved to go in breads and cookies. How about those celery ends and leaves? Perfect for the stock pot.

By using everything, you save money, the environment, and it all just tastes so good.

DON'T BE AFRAID TO TRY

Just because most people don't do it anymore, doesn't mean it's hard. It just means that "most people" don't make the time, don't have the time, or don't really know it exists. Take canning, for example. We are about two generations away from home-canned goods being a regular kitchen staple.

My grandmother canned most of her own vegetables and fruits. My parents even canned tomatoes, beans, and jams. Industrialization of our food supply has made it so convenient to pick stuff up at the store rather than making it ourselves, but we're also picking up lots of additives, sugar, fats, and things that aren't really food in our manufactured aluminum cans.

Slow down, relax, and make canning, dehydrating, baking, and slow-cooking an enjoyable experience. You are nourishing your body and the bodies of the people you love. Make it wonderful.

BIG BATCHES
MAKE ANOTHER DAY EASIER

When you're preparing something in the kitchen, whether it's a roast for dinner or cookies for the kids, make big batches. That way, you can freeze or wrap leftovers for those days when you're just too busy to even catch your breath.

Make two loaves of bread instead of one. Wrap one really tightly and freeze it for several weeks. If it's for sandwiches, pre-slice it so it can be used straight out of the freezer! You can also freeze butter, cookies, biscuits, scones, meats, gravies, and many casseroles.

If you're making almond meal for cookies, make extra and store it in a glass jar so you don't need to get out your food processor the next time you need some. This simple tip has often meant the difference between me being motivated to make dessert and not. (I don't like to wash dishes.)

The following recipes are homemade versions of things you might buy at the grocery store, or they're easily freezable or storable recipes that are great to have on hand. Of course there's the canning, which I really hope you try. Just when you thought food couldn't get more real. This is real human food for real humans, made from the scratchiest scratch you can get.

HOW TO CAN
WITH A HOT WATER BATH

Let me start out by saying, don't be afraid! Canning can be simple, fun, and even relaxing! All you need is a big pot, some canning tongs, jars, lids, and rims, and you're equipped! Well, and something to put into those jars, of course.

Just to be clear, not every fruit and vegetable can be preserved with a hot water bath canning technique. Some need a pressure canner. But the recipes here are easily canned (jam, fruit, pickles and tomatoes) in a hot water bath, and are perfect for beginners and seasoned canners alike!

Here's the basic hot water bath canning method.

Supplies:

- Canning Pot or Large Stock Pot
- Jar lifters (canning tongs)
- Clean jars, new lids, and rings
- Canning Funnel
- Towels and pot holders
- Food to be canned and anything necessary to prep it

Process:

Your food has to be hot to use this canning method. So if it's going to take longer for your product to process (tomato sauce, applesauce), you should get that cooking first.

Your jars must be warm when they are filled. The best method is to wash the jars in the dishwasher with the heated drying option turned on. If you time it properly, the jars will be done washing when you need them, and can stay in the closed dishwasher staying warm for a bit until you're ready.

Your seals must also be warm. Place the seals (lids) into a pan of water and bring to a boil. Remove from heat, but keep them in the water until you're ready to use them.

Fill your pot about ¾ full of water and bring to just under a boil. Prepare your food according to the recipe. When it's piping hot, pour it into the clean, hot jars using a canning funnel. Fill to recommended fill line, usually just at the bottom of the ring threads.

Use a small rubber spatula to remove any bubbles in the filled jars by sliding it down the inside edges. Wipe the rims clean and dry with a paper towel.

Place the seals and rings onto the filled jars, tightening until snug. Bring the water to a low boil. Place the jars down into the canning rack. If you're using regular stock pot, you'll want to put something in it to keep the jars off the bottom, such as a hand towel or block. It's best to use the canning pot with rack because it also prevents the jars from knocking into one another.

Boil for recommended time (adjusted for altitude), making sure the water is completely covering the jars. When time is up, remove the jars with the tongs to a butcher block or a thick towel. Make sure you leave an inch or so between jars.

Do not touch the lids at this point. They haven't sealed yet and you could ruin all of your effort. Keep the kids away, too!

Now, listen carefully. You'll start to hear the lids pop! When the jars are completely cooled, you can press on the lids. The lids should be sucked down. If a jar is still popped up, then it's not sealed and you'll have to put that one into the fridge to eat within the next few days. Always label your jars with the contents and the date. Store in a cool, dark place.

HOT WATER BATH CANNING

HONEY PEARS
DILL PICKLES
CINNAMON APPLESAUCE
MARINARA SAUCE

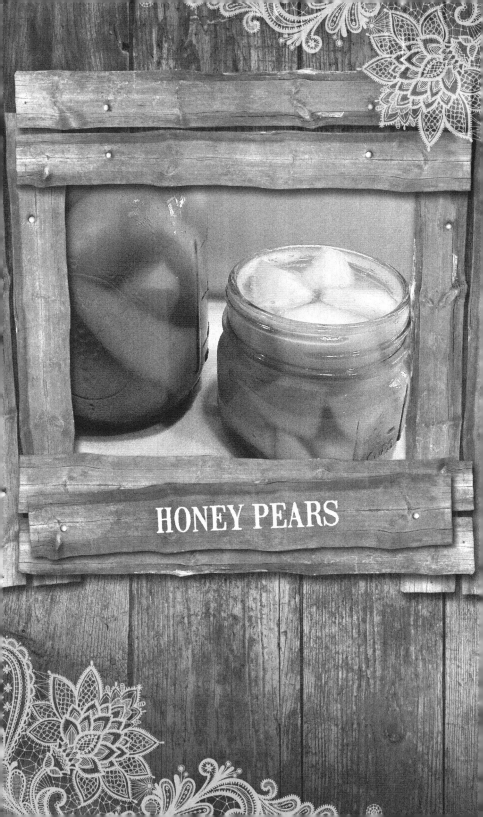

HONEY PEARS

HONEY PEARS, OR KIDS WITH BRACES

My son has braces. I see him every day, and yet that concept escapes me when I pack his lunch. When he comes home with his apple or pear still in his lunch box, I realize why. He can't eat the crisp fruit! Now, he loves these honey-canned pears and always comes home with an empty jar!

This recipe varies based on how many pears you want to can. I'm giving you the basics, so you can do a bushel or a quart, depending on your level of ambition!

HONEY PEARS RECIPE

Ingredients:

- Fresh pears, not too ripe
- Lemon juice
- Raw honey
- Pure filtered water
- Canning jars, lids, and rings

Directions: Peel the pears and cut them into your desired shape. Fill your jars to 1" from the top with pears. Add one tablespoon of lemon juice to the pears to prevent browning.

Bring a solution of 1 ½ cups honey to 4 cups water (1.5 honey : 4 water) to a rolling boil. Pour the honey syrup over the tops of the jarred pears, filling to 1" below the jar rim.

Can according to hot water bath instructions.

Hot water bath boiling time for pears is 15- 20 minutes for pints and 20 -25 minutes for quarts.

Serving Size: 1 cup   Yields: Varies
Prep Time: 30 min – hours, depending on your quantity

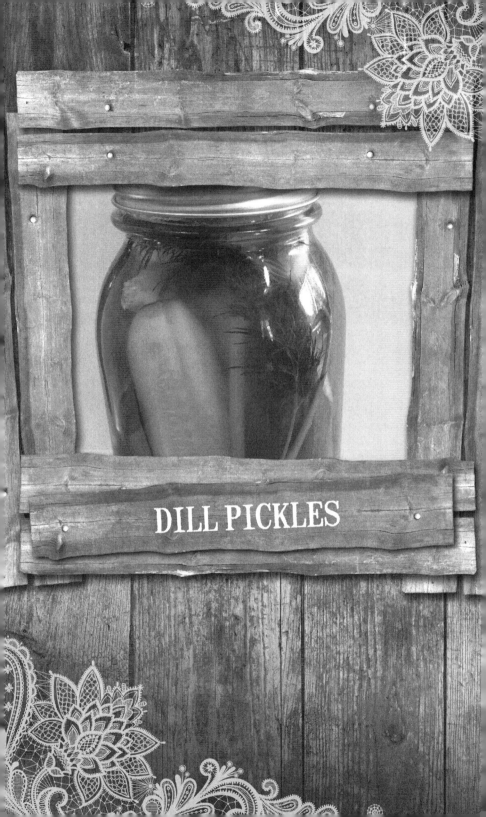

DILL PICKLES

DILL PICKLES, OR A TASTE OF SUMMER!

I'm not a master gardener, but I do have a little patch in my back yard where a few things grow if I'm lucky. One thing that I always manage to harvest is cucumber. A lot of cucumber. So my family has taken to making pickles so we can enjoy the fruits of our labor all year round. Our favorite is garlic dill, but you can make the pickles with spicy peppers if you like a little kick!

DILL PICKLE RECIPE

Ingredients:

- 50 – 60 baby cucumbers (or pickle cucumbers)
- 8 cups white vinegar
- 4 cups filtered water
- 1 cup sea salt
- 10 pint jars
- 10 large sprigs fresh dill
- 20 garlic cloves, peeled

Directions: Bring the water, vinegar, and salt to a boil in a large pot. Wash the cucumbers and slice them in half vertically (or can whole). Distribute the cucumbers into the jars, leaving about an inch of space at the top. Add one sprig of dill and two cloves of garlic to each jar.

Pour the boiling vinegar mixture over the tops of the cucumber, filling the jar to about 1" from the top. Place lids and rings on the jars and process with the hot water bath canning method.

Hot water bath boiling time for pickles is 15 minutes.

Serving Size: 2 pickles   Yields: Varies/ about 50 servings
Prep Time: 30 min   Canning Time: 30 min
Total Time: 60 min

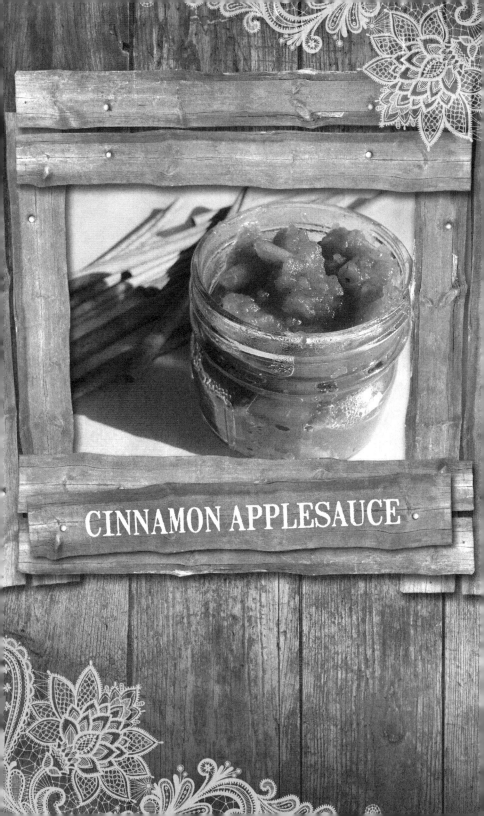

CINNAMON APPLESAUCE

CINNAMON APPLESAUCE, OR MY PRIDE AND JOY

I love applesauce. It's nature's sweet dessert with the benefit of being healthy and simple to make. I can this in small jars so it can go straight into my kids' lunch boxes, where they gloat over their applesauce next to the other kids' plastic containers.

CINNAMON APPLESAUCE RECIPE

Ingredients:

- Apples, any variety and any quantity
- Ground cinnamon
- Filtered water

Directions: Peel and core the apples. Cut them into large chunks and place them into a big heavy pot set over low heat. Add about 1 teaspoon of cinnamon for every four apples and enough water so the apples don't burn to the bottom. Stir regularly, simmering the apples for 15 – 30 minutes (depending on quantity) until they are cooked and mushy.
Scoop the applesauce into prepared canning jars and can according to hot water bath canning instructions.

Hot water bath boiling time for applesauce is 12 minutes for 4-oz jars, 15 minutes for pint jars, and 20 minutes for quart jars.

Serving Size: ½ cup   Yields: Varies
Prep Time: 20 min +   Canning Time: 12 min+

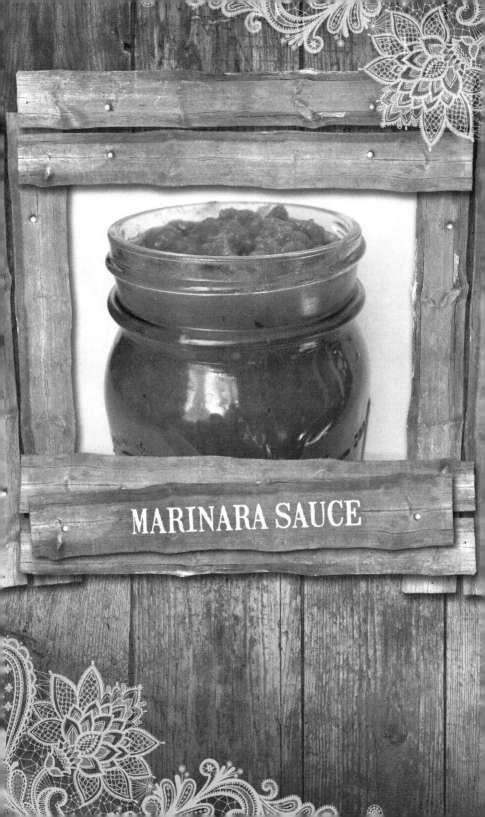

MARINARA SAUCE

MARINARA SAUCE,
OR WHAT MY DAUGHTER EATS

Sometimes my daughter is an adventurous eater, other times she isn't. But the one thing I can always get her to eat is marinara sauce. We bake it with eggplant, pour it over spaghetti squash, or even eat it like stew mixed with sautéed ground meats and veggies. When tomatoes are ripe, you can stock up your pantry with this healthy staple for very little cost.

MARINARA SAUCE RECIPE

Ingredients:

- 5 lb fresh tomatoes
- 10 oz tomato paste
- 4 Garlic cloves, minced
- 1 White onion, finely chopped
- 3 tbsp olive oil
- 2 tbsp chopped fresh oregano
- 2 tbsp chopped fresh basil
- 2 tbsp honey or birch xylitol
- 3 tsp sea salt
- ½ cup red wine vinegar (necessary for canning)
- ½ tsp black pepper
- ½ tsp red pepper flakes
- ½ cup chicken broth

Directions: Place tomatoes and tomato paste in the food processor and process until smooth. In a large pot or Dutch oven, sauté the garlic and onion in olive oil until translucent and fragrant. Add remaining ingredients, stir, and simmer on low for about 1 ½ hours. Sauce will be darker, richer, and the liquids will be reduced. Add 1 tablespoon lemon juice to pint jars and 2 tablespoons to quart jars before canning. This is necessary to lower the pH to below 4.5 to make it safe for hot water bath canning. Otherwise, botulism can grow, making the sauce unsafe.

Can in clean jars according to the hot water bath method. This recipe only makes 80 ounces of sauce, but is easily doubled or tripled or more! Hot water bath processing time for tomato sauce is 35 minutes for pint jars and 45 minutes for quart jars.

Serving Size: 1 cup   Yields: about 7 servings   Prep Time: 10 minutes
Cook Time: 1 ½ hours   Canning Time: 45 min

CHILLED OUT

BLACKBERRY FREEZER JAM
HAZELNUT ICE BOX COOKIES
BANANA BLISS ICE CREAM
HAPPY CHICKEN NUGGETS
SAUERKRAUT

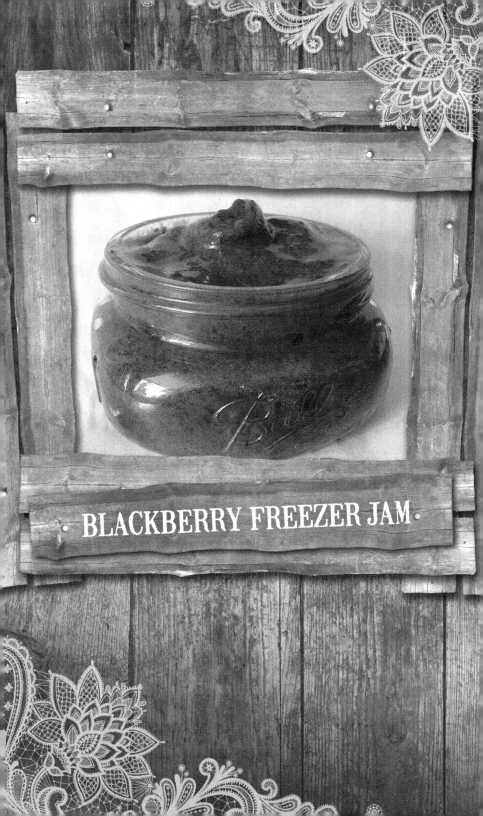

BLACKBERRY FREEZER JAM

BLACKBERRY FREEZER JAM, OR YOU CAN'T TOP THIS

You can't top this blackberry jam, but it can top just about anything! Perfect on Paleo toast or scones, waffles, pancakes, and even on steak! While traditional jam is full of sugar, this one uses pure honey and a little guar gum for thickener. That's it. All you taste is pure, natural goodness.

BLACKBERRY FREEZER JAM

Ingredients:

- 2 cups fresh or frozen blackberries
- 2 tsp raw honey (or to taste)
- ½ tsp guar gum (or 1 tsp tapioca starch, if you're not using guar)

Directions: Place all ingredients in the food processor and process until smooth. Pour into jars with tight-fitting lids and freeze up to three months. This jam stays good in the refrigerator up to two weeks.

Serving Size: 2 tbsp   Yields: about 10 servings
Prep Time: 5 min   Total Time: 5 min

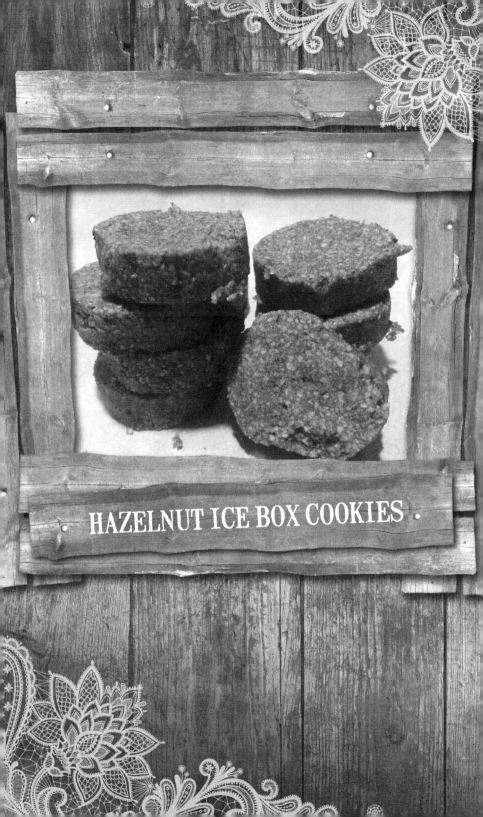

HAZELNUT ICE BOX COOKIES

HAZELNUT ICE BOX COOKIES, OR SURPRISE GUESTS

You get that knock on the door, and it's your neighbor who just showed up for coffee and conversation! You can be prepared by keeping this delicious cookie dough in your freezer at all times. It's the perfect bite to go with your coffee or tea... or almond milk... or anything!

HAZELNUT ICE BOX COOKIE RECIPE

Ingredients:

- 2 cups hazelnut meal
- 3 tbsp coconut oil
- 2 tbsp raw honey
- 2 tbsp cocoa powder
- ½ tsp vanilla
- ½ tsp baking soda

Directions: Place all ingredients in a large bowl and beat with electric beaters until a dough ball forms, about two minutes.

Pour the dough-ball out on a sheet of waxed paper and roll into about an 8 – 10" log. Flatten the ends and roll the whole thing in waxed paper. Place the waxed paper into a plastic bag, lidded container, or another layer of waxed paper and freeze until ready to use.

For baking: Preheat the oven to 325°F. Remove the cookie dough from the freezer and slice into ½" rounds. Lay the rounds on a parchment-lined cookie sheet and bake in the preheated oven for 12 – 15 minutes or until crisp.

Serving Size: 2 cookies   Yields: 8 servings
Prep Time: 10 min   Bake Time: 15 min   Total Time: 25 min

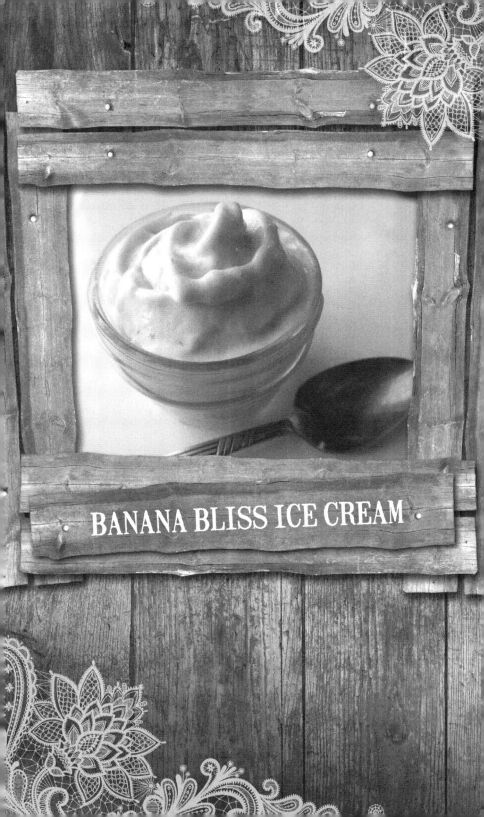

BANANA BLISS ICE CREAM

BANANA BLISS ICE CREAM, OR SILLY EASY CREAMY BEST ICE CREAM EVER!

One of my vices in switching to Paleo, especially after having 'One-of-those-days' was ice cream. I was a Hagen-o-holic, and for obvious reasons, I knew I needed to come up with a healthier alternative. There are some knock-off recipes in Paleo that can leave you feeling less than satisfied, but this is NOT one of them. This recipe is so simple. It's one ingredient, and beyond easy to whip up - even in your weakest moments. It's also an excellent way to use up those bananas that are a little on the too ripe side so you don't have to toss them.

BANANA BLISS ICE CREAM RECIPE

Ingredients:

- 2 frozen ripe bananas (make sure to freeze them without the peel)

Optional add-ons:

- Seeds from 1/2 vanilla bean (or 1/2 teaspoon vanilla extract)
- 1 tablespoon maple syrup/date paste
- 1 1/3 tbsp dark cocoa powder
- Other frozen fruit
- Chilled espresso
- 1 tbsp almond butter
- Or any combination thereof

Directions: Put everything into your high-powered blender and blend until it is super smooth, like vanilla soft serve. Make sure you keep pushing the bananas down into the blades. If you find your blender isn't blending the mix well you can add 1/4 cup or less (watch for consistency) almond milk. Serve with desired toppings, or eat straight out of the blender (or is that just me?).

Serving size 3/4 cup   Yield : 2 servings (or 1 very hungry serving)
Prep Time: 5 min   Mix Time: 5 min   Total Time 10 min

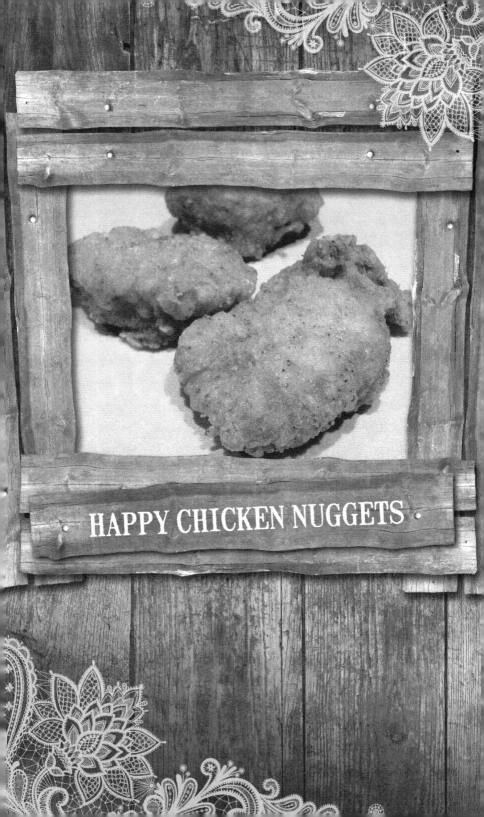

HAPPY CHICKEN NUGGETS

HAPPY CHICKEN NUGGETS, OR EAT SOMETHING, PLEASE!

My children have friends. This is a problem on insomuch as that many of their friends do not eat a healthy diet, and won't even try the delicious and wholesome foods we have around our house. That's where having a bag of these chicken nuggets stashed in the freezer really comes in handy! I just pull a few out, pop them in the toaster oven, and serve them up with a little ramekin of raw honey or honey-mustard. Finally, I can get those crazy kids to eat something!

HAPPY CHICKEN NUGGETS RECIPE

Ingredients:

- 2 lbs bones, skinless chicken breast
- 2 Eggs, beaten
- 1 ½ cups tapioca starch
- 1 pint avocado oil
- ½ tsp each: garlic powder, paprika, sea salt, ground black pepper

Directions: Set the oil in a medium-sized heavy saucepan set over high heat, or in a deep fryer.

Cut the chicken into nugget-sized pieces. In a large bowl, combine tapioca starch and spices and mix well. Beat the eggs in another bowl.

Dunk the chicken nuggets first into the flour, then into the egg wash, then back into the flour mixture. This will give them a nice thick coating that sticks! Drop the coated nuggets into the hot oil in small batches. Cook for about five minutes (depending on size of pieces), turning once during cooking to ensure an even cook.

Remove with a slatted spoon to a paper-towel lined plate. Once the nuggets are cooled, you can place them in a single layer in an airtight container or zipper bag and freeze for later.

To Reheat: Remove the desired quantity of nuggets from the freezer and place directly on a baking sheet. Bake in a preheated 375° F oven or toaster oven for 5 – 10 minutes or until warmed through and crisp.

Serving Size: 5 nuggets   Yields: 4 servings
Prep Time: About 20 min   Bake Time (from frozen): **5 – 10 min**

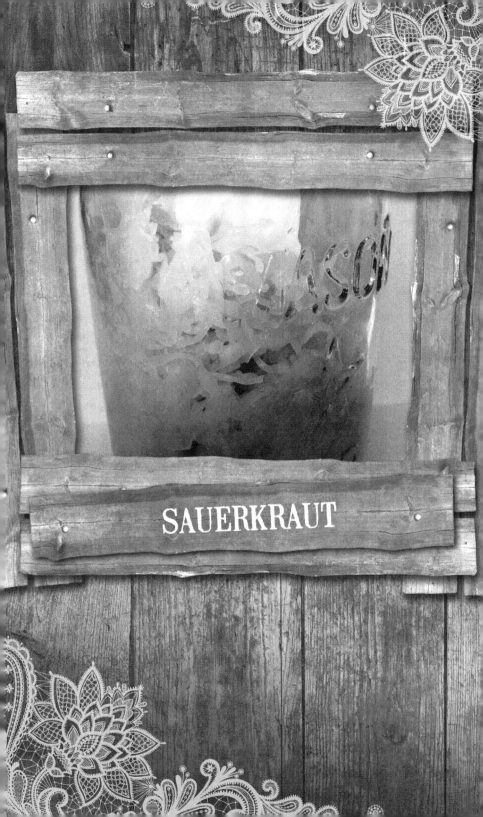

SAUERKRAUT

SAUERKRAUT, OR NOW I UNDERSTAND

As a kid, I hated sauerkraut. I hated the smell and the texture and I couldn't understand why anyone would ruin a perfectly good sausage by dousing it with this stuff. But now I'm older, and wiser. I not only love sauerkraut for its flavor, but for the gut-healing properties of this fermented food. Sauerkraut, I finally understand you.

SAUERKRAUT RECIPE

Ingredients:

- 1 ½ lbs green cabbage
- ½ tsp kosher salt

Directions: Quarter and core the cabbage. With a large, sharp knife, slice the cabbage into very thin strips and place them in a large bowl. Sprinkle the cabbage with the salt.

Now's where the fun begins. Dig in there with your hands (washed, of course) and squeeze the cabbage. Or, you can mash it with a potato masher. Either way, the goal is to get the cabbage to release its juices.

Once the cabbage is quite wet, scrape it into a wide-mouthed glass jar or ceramic kraut pot. Place a small, heavy plate (or some other type of broad weight) on top of the cabbage and press down to release some more of the juices. Leave the weight there, and throw a clean towel or piece of cloth over the top of the jar. Store it in a cool part of your kitchen.

Check on your kraut every few hours that first day, pressing down on the weight each time to release juices. In 24 hours, if the brine isn't fully covering the cabbage, add a saltwater solution (1 tsp salt to 1 cup water) to bring that liquid up over the top.

Keep checking on your kraut over the next few days. It should be bubbling and a white scum will form on the top. Scrape off the scum... but don't worry, that means it's working! Taste your kraut every three days or so. Stop when you like the flavor! You can ferment it up to 10 days, at which point you should scrape it into glass jars and store it in the refrigerator for up to two months.

Serving Size: 1 cup   Yields: about 4 servings (1 quart)
Prep Time: 15 min   Ferment Time: 10 days

THE BASICS

MEALS & FLOURS
ALMOND BUTTER
GRASS-FED BUTTER
SPREADABLE WHIPPED BUTTER BLEND
HOMEMADE BEEF BROTH
HOMEMADE CHICKEN BROTH
CREAMY SOUP MIX
DRIED CHERRIES

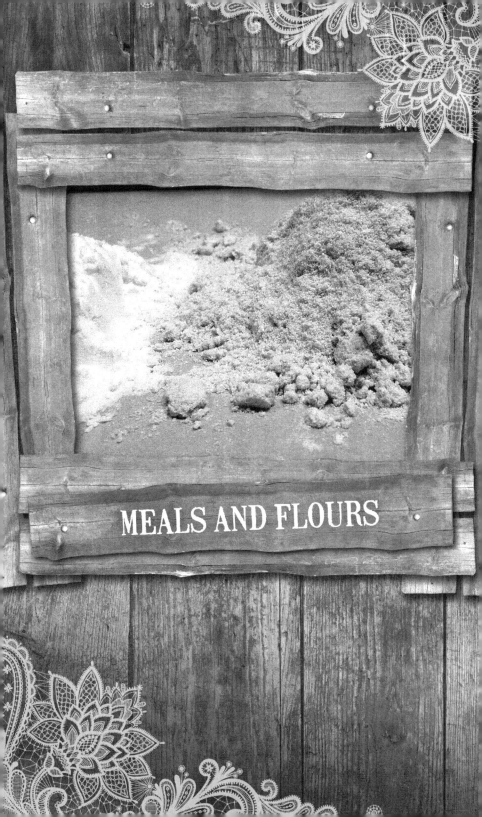

MEALS AND FLOURS

FLOURS, NUTMEALS, AND STARCHES,
OR WHERE DO I GET THAT?

Sometimes a friend will ask me, "Where do you buy coconut flour?" Or, "Hazelnut meal? My grocery store doesn't have it." The answer is in the kitchen appliance. If your local market doesn't carry coconut flour, make it yourself out of unsweetened shredded coconut by tossing it into your food processor or, even better, your high-powered blender (like a Vitamix).

 Since these flours and meals are the mainstay of a Paleo kitchen, especially if you like to bake, it's important to know your way around them. Meals are grainier and oilier than flours, while starches are the lightest and smoothest for baked goods and thickening sauces. Making your own really allows for diversity and creativity in your baking. How about pistachio meal for a new cookie recipe? Maybe dried-yam flour for making bread? The possibilities are nearly endless.

FLOUR, NUTMEAL, AND STARCH DIRECTIONS

I feel a little silly calling this a recipe, so I didn't. I called it "directions." All you do is start out with the ingredient you want to turn into a meal, flour, or starch.

For example:

- Dried coconut
- Almonds (raw, blanched, or with skin)
- Cashews
- Hazelnuts
- Tapioca (starch)
- Macadamia nuts
- Pecans
- Walnuts

Place any quantity of the ingredient into the blender and process until it resembles the coarseness of flour or meal you require. It's important to stop at some point during the process to push down any flyaway pieces with a rubber spatula so you end up with an even consistency. Just watch carefully, because if you blend it too long it will turn into butter (almond butter, etc).

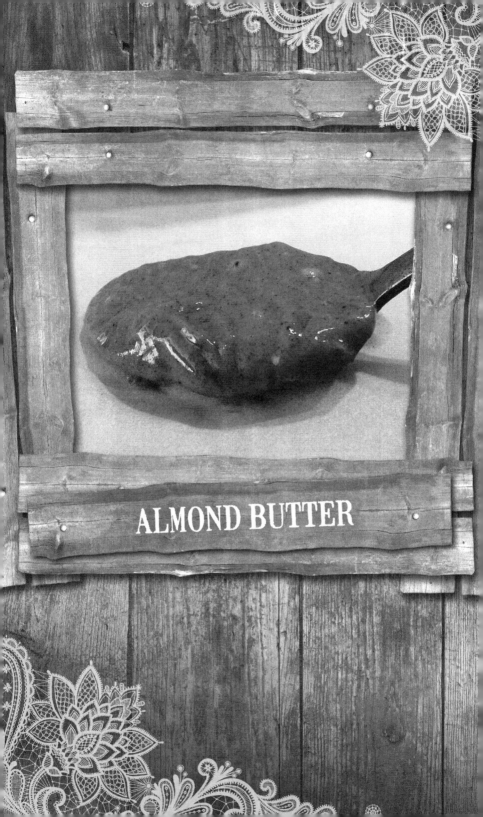

ALMOND BUTTER

ALMOND BUTTER, OR YOU'RE NUTS!

Yes, I make my own almond butter... and macadamia nut butter, and cashew butter, and even some cocoa-hazelnut butter that tastes a bit like Nutella! Am I nuts? Yes, I'm nuts about nuts! And making the nut butter at home is good for several reasons. It's easy, it's healthy, and I don't have to have as many things in my pantry. I can buy one big bag of almonds and have nuts, meal, flour, milk, and butter from that single purchase.

ALMOND BUTTER RECIPE

Ingredients:

- 2 cups raw almonds
- 2 tsp raw honey
- 1 tsp coconut oil
- ½ tsp sea salt

Directions: Preheat the oven to 350°F. Spread your almonds in an even layer on a rimmed baking sheet. Roast in the preheated oven for about eight minutes. Using oven mitts, grasp the pan and give the nuts a good shake. Return to the oven and roast an additional eight to ten minutes. Use your nose. If you can smell them, and they smell roasted, they're done!

Remove the pan from the oven and let the nuts cool a little bit so they're easier to work with. Once slightly cooled, place the nuts into your food processor. Process until smooth, scraping down the sides when necessary.

While the almond butter is now done, I like to add a bit of flavor to mine. Add the coconut oil, honey, and sea salt to the smooth nut butter and process for a few more seconds to incorporate.

Pour the almond butter into a clean glass jar with a tight-fitting lid and store in the refrigerator for up to three months.

Serving Size: 2 tablespoons   Yields: about 20 servings
Prep Time: 5 min   Bake Time: 18 min   Total Time: 23 min

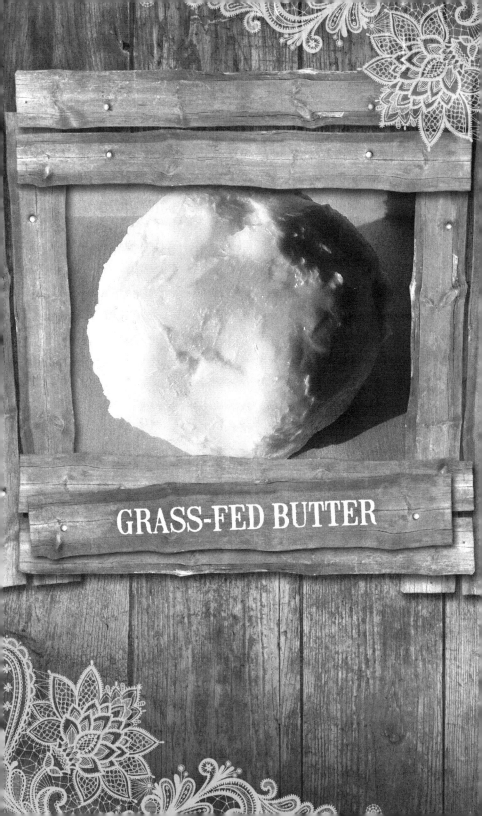

GRASS-FED BUTTER

GRASS-FED BUTTER, OR PURE GOODNESS

Nothing, and I mean nothing tastes better than fresh home-churned butter. No, I don't have a butter churn in my kitchen. But I do have a standing mixer, which we found out was much more efficient than shaking the cream in a mason jar... Try rolling a knob of your butter in fresh chopped herbs and bringing it out at your next dinner party! Seriously, forget about a cheese ball! We Paleos go straight for the butterball!

GRASS-FED BUTTER DIRECTIONS

Ingredients:

- 1 quart fresh grass-fed heavy cream (local if possible)
- Salt, if desired

Directions: Place the cold cream into the bowl of your standing mixer fixed with a whisk attachment. Turn it on to medium-high speed.

Walk away, wash your dishes, read a book. The butter will make itself. Within about fifteen minutes, the cream will begin to get slushy, then it will froth. Next it will turn into whipped cream. Then it will turn into firm whipped cream, and suddenly it will curd and you'll hear it sloshing. Watch it now, because it will quickly clump up into a yellow ball of butter!

At this point, pour off the buttermilk and add ½ cup or so of ice water and salt (if using). Turn on the beater again for a few seconds until the wash water is milky. Pour it off and repeat about three times until the wash water comes out clear.

Place the butterball into a mason jar with a lid and shake to release any excess moisture. Pour it off and do it again, a couple of times until the butterball is clean and "dry." Store it in a glass jar in the refrigerator up to two weeks, or freeze for up to two months.

Serving Size: 1 ounce   Yields: 16 servings (one pound)
Prep Time: 30 min   Total Time: 30 min

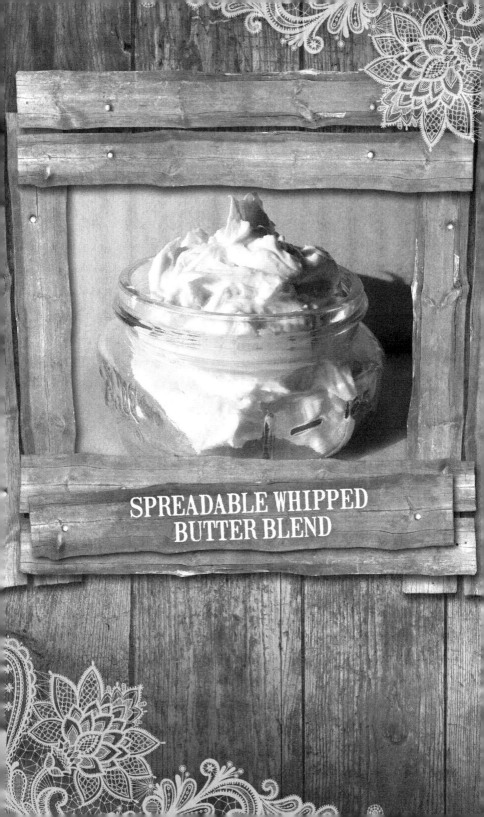

SPREADABLE WHIPPED
BUTTER BLEND

SPREADABLE WHIPPED BUTTER BLEND, OR I CAN'T BELIEVE IT'S NOT HARD!

This whipped spread is the perfect balance of heart-healthy avocado oil and delicious fresh grass-fed butter. But more importantly, it's soft straight from the fridge! Spread it right onto your almond roll, muffin, or sweet potato pancake without tearing giant holes in your food. Your children will thank you for it.

SPREADABLE WHIPPED BUTTER BLEND RECIPE

Ingredients:

- ½ cup fresh grass-fed butter, softened
- ½ cup avocado or olive oil

Directions: Place the butter and oil in a large mixing bowl or standing mixer. Beat on high until light and fluffy, about two minutes. Store in a glass jar in the refrigerator up to two weeks... if you down gobble it all up by then!

Serving Size: 1 ounce   Yields: 16 servings
Prep Time: 5 min   Total Time: 5 min

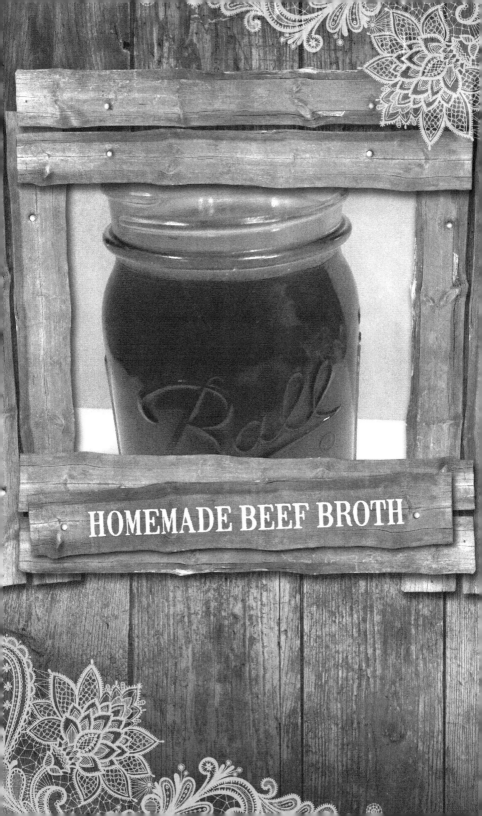

HOMEMADE BEEF BROTH

BEEF BROTH, OR SOUP'S ON!

A hot meal is just a jar away when you keep your fridge and freezer stocked with broth. Pour it into a pot with some diced veggies, herbs and spices and you can feed a hungry army in minutes! I never throw away a bone from beef, pork, or chicken. The bones go straight into my slow cooker where they turn water into a delicious base for soups and gravies.

BEEF BROTH RECIPE

Ingredients:

- 7 - 10 Beef bones left over from steaks or roasts (cooked, with marrow)
- 2 Onions
- 2 Carrots
- Handful fresh parsley
- 3 Cloves garlic
- 1 tbsp peppercorns
- 1 tsp sea salt
- Filtered water to cover, about four quarts

Directions: Place the bones in the bottom of a large slow cooker. Peel and quarter the onions. Scrub the carrots and cut to fit pot. Peel the garlic. Place all the vegetables and seasoning in the pot and cover with water. You can fill your slow cooker up to about an inch from the top.

Simmer in the slow cooker on low for about 24 hours. Allow to cool enough for you to handle, and then pour the broth through a fine mesh sieve into any size glass mason jars. Store it in the refrigerator up to a week.

Once it's completely cooled, you can freeze it up to three months. However, you may want to transfer to BPA-free plastic containers to reduce risk of cracking.

Serving Size: 1 cup   Yields: about 5 quarts
Prep Time: 15 min   Cook Time: 24 hours
Total Time: 24 hrs 15 min

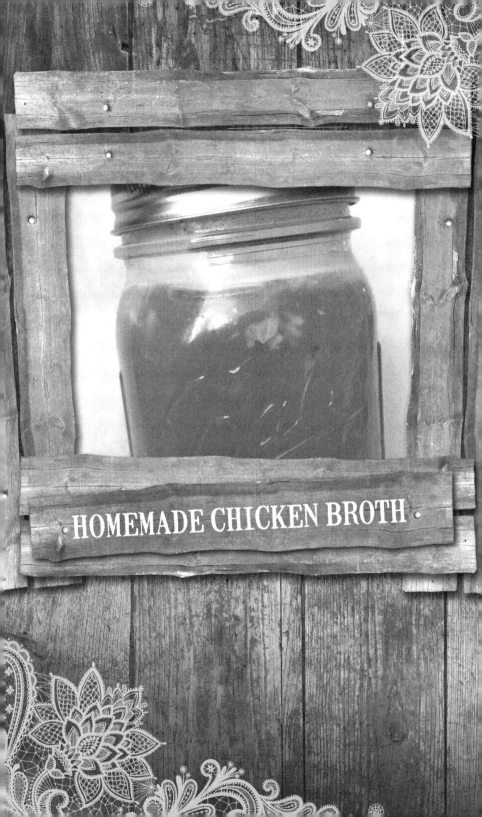

HOMEMADE CHICKEN BROTH

CHICKEN BROTH,
OR IT SMELLS LIKE GRANDMA'S HOUSE!

When you walk into a house that has chicken broth simmering in the crock-pot, it makes you feel warm and loved... just like the smell of grandma's slow-cooked chicken soup. No bit of the chicken goes to waste in our house. As soon as our family is done enjoying a roasted chicken dinner, the carcass goes into the slow cooker with veggies and seasonings. Try it, and you'll never pay for prepackaged broth again!

CHICKEN BROTH RECIPE

Ingredients:

- 1 Roasted chicken carcass
- 1 Onion, peeled and quartered
- 2 Small carrots, scrubbed
- 2 Celery stalks, washed
- 2 Bay leaves
- 10 Peppercorns
- 2 tsp sea salt
- 4 quarts filtered water, or to cover

Directions: Place the chicken carcass and all of the vegetables and spices into the slow cooker. Pour water over the top to cover. You can fill your slow cooker up to about one inch from the top. Simmer on low for 24 hours. Allow to cool enough to handle.

Pour the broth through a fine sieve into glass quart jars. Store in the refrigerator for up to one week, or transfer to BPA-free plastic containers and freeze up to three months. Use this broth for soups, gravies, and casseroles.

Serving Size: 1 cup   Yields: about 4 quarts   Prep Time: 10 min
Cook Time: 24 hours   Total Time: 24 hrs 10 min

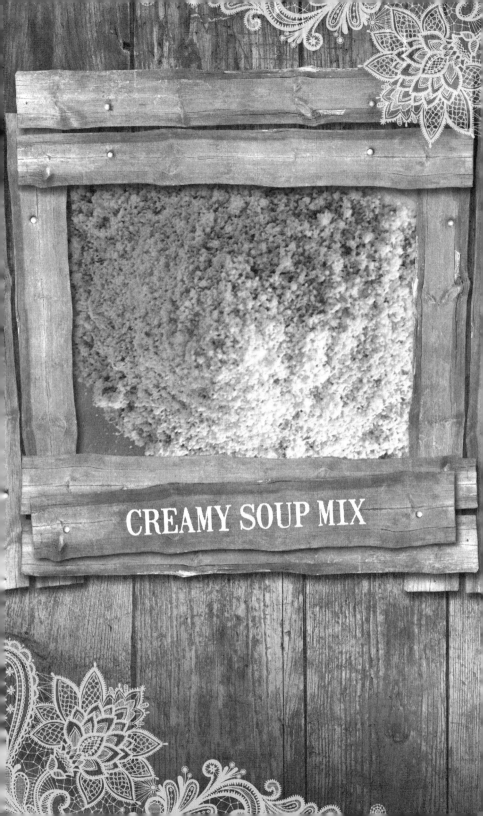

CREAMY SOUP MIX

CREAMY SOUP MIX
OR S.O.S. SAVE MY SANITY MIX
(REPLACEMENT TO CANNED CREAMED SOUPS)

This frugal make ahead and store recipe can be used as a replacement for creamed soups in any recipe, as well as the base for other sauces, gravies, soups and much more including the delicious Cream of Mushroom Soup recipe (see recipe on page 77). This is a bulk recipe and makes the equivalent to 9 cans of cream soup.

PALEO SOUP OR SAUCE MIX

Ingredients:

- 2 cups of almond meal
- ¾ cup of arrowroot flour
- 2 tbsp dried onion flakes
- 2 tsp of Italian Seasoning or a combination of dried Parsley, Oregano and Basil
- 1 tsp of black pepper

Directions: Combine all of the above dry ingredients and stir until blended.

Store in a Ziploc, glass or plastic jar or even a can to use when needed. It can be stored on the shelf! Or refrigerate for extra freshness.

Instructions to substitute for 1-10.75 oz can of creamed soup:

Combine ⅓ cup of dry mix with 1¼ cups of chicken or beef broth. Cook and stir on the stovetop until thickened. Add thickened mixture to the casseroles/recipes just as you would a can of soup.

Yield: This amount is equal to using (9) 10.75 cans of creamed soups
Prep time: 5 min   Total time: 5 min
Serves: Equal to 9 cans of cream soup

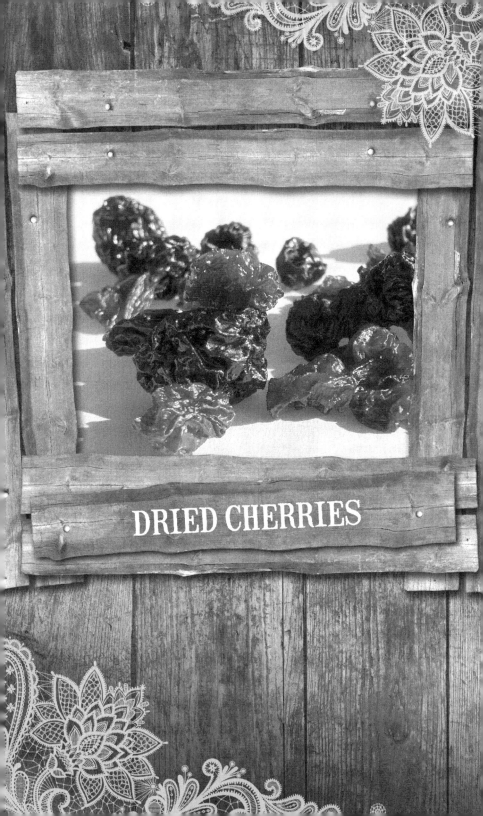

DRIED CHERRIES

DRIED CHERRIES, OR ANY BERRY, REALLY

Once you realize how simple it is to dry a cherry (which I know isn't a berry), you'll never buy them again. I was making a recipe for energy bars when I realized that I didn't have the dried cherries on hand. The store closest to me didn't have any without added sugar, so I picked up a bag of frozen cherries instead. This happened to be a blend of dark sweet cherries and their smaller, tarter cousin, the bing cherry. You can even use this oven method to dry blueberries, grapes, plums, and even strawberries!

DRIED CHERRY DIRECTIONS

Ingredients:

- 2 cups frozen or fresh pitted cherries

Directions: Preheat oven to 170°F. Spread the cherries on a wire rack set into a jellyroll pan. Bake in the prepared oven for about ten hours, or until the juices have evaporated and the fruit is shriveled.

Serving Size: 2 tablespoons   Yields: about 8 servings
Prep Time: 5 min   Bake Time: 10 hours   Total Time: 10 hrs 5 min

SNACKS AND DRINKS

LEMONADE
TERIYAKI BEEF JERKY
HONEY ROASTED ALMONDS
APPLE CHIPS
PLANTAIN CHIPS
COOKIE DOUGH BITES

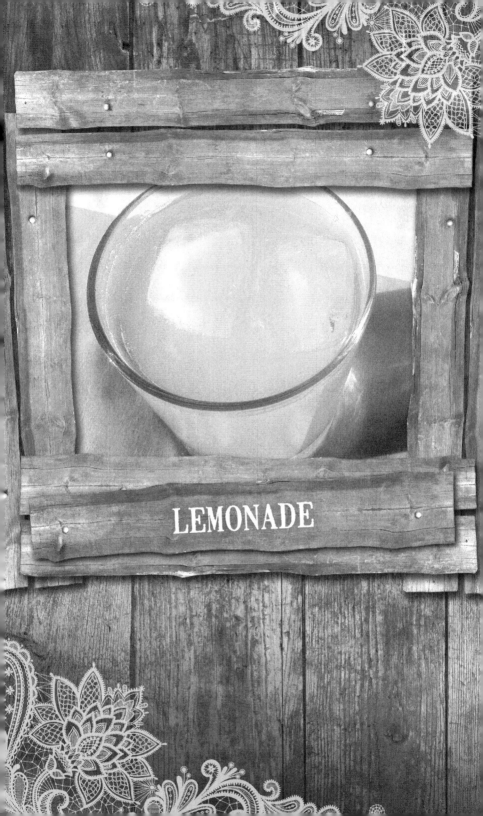

LEMONADE

LEMONADE, OR SIMPLE PLEASURES

My children love summer! One of their favorite things to do is have a lemonade stand, but I don't have the traditional bag of sugar or can of mix sitting in my cupboard. So we came up with this delicious, Paleo-friendly alternative that sweetens the tart lemon juice with fresh apple juice and honey. We use our juicer (I'm in love with kitchen appliances), but you could substitute natural apple juice in this recipe.

LEMONADE RECIPE

Ingredients:

- 1 cup freshly squeezed lemon juice
- 1 cup juice from freshly juiced Golden Delicious apples
- ¾ cups raw honey (or to taste)
- 2 quarts filtered water

Directions: Pour the honey into the bottom of a large pitcher. Bring one cup of the water to a simmer and pour it over the honey. Stir until the honey is all melted with no clumps. Allow to cool slightly, then add the lemon and Golden Delicious apple juices. Stir and fill the rest of the pitcher with ice.

Serving Size: 1 cup   Yields: 11 servings
Prep Time: 5 min   (plus juicing)   Total Time: 5-10 min

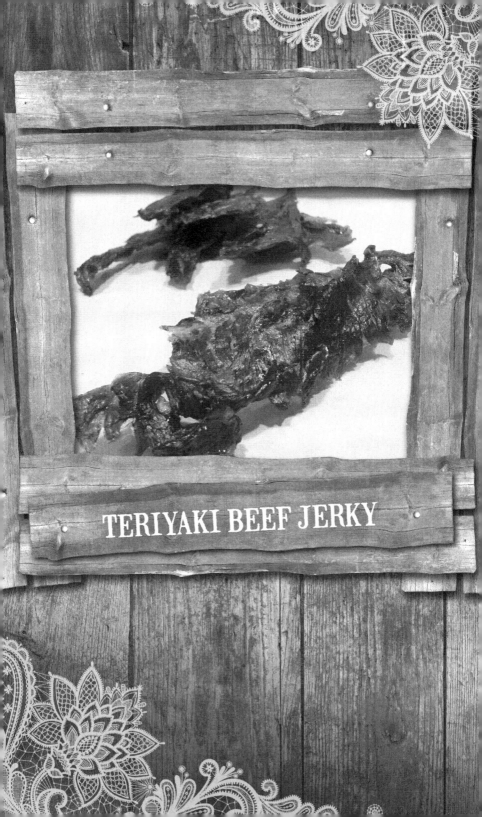

TERIYAKI BEEF JERKY

TERIYAKI BEEF JERKY,
OR FEEDING TEENAGE BOYS

Beef jerky is a go-to snack in our house. It's full of protein and its chewy, savory goodness is adored by everyone... especially my teenage son and his friends! Sometimes I think they're going to eat me out of house and home! Unfortunately, it's hard to find jerky in the store that doesn't have sugar or nitrites among a host of other additives. Good thing it's so easy to make your own!

TERIYAKI BEEF JERKY RECIPE

Ingredients:

- 1 lb flank steak
- ¼ cup pure maple syrup
- ¼ cup liquid coconut aminos
- 1 tsp crushed garlic
- Black pepper to taste

Directions: Trim the fat from the flank steak. With a sharp knife, slice the steak against the grain into very thin slices. Place the meat and all remaining ingredients into a large zip-top bag or container and shake to coat. Let the meat marinade overnight.

Preheat oven to 175°F. Place a wire rack on top of a jelly roll pan and lay the marinated meat sliced in a single layer on the rack, making sure the pieces do not touch. Bake for 8 – 12 hours (depending on thickness of cut) until all the moisture is out of the meat and the jerky is chewy, but not crispy.

Store in an airtight container in the cupboard for up to ten days or refrigerate for up to three weeks.

Serving Size: 3 pieces   Yields: about 5 servings
Prep Time: 5 min plus overnight   Bake Time: 8 – 12 hours
Total Time: 1 ½ days

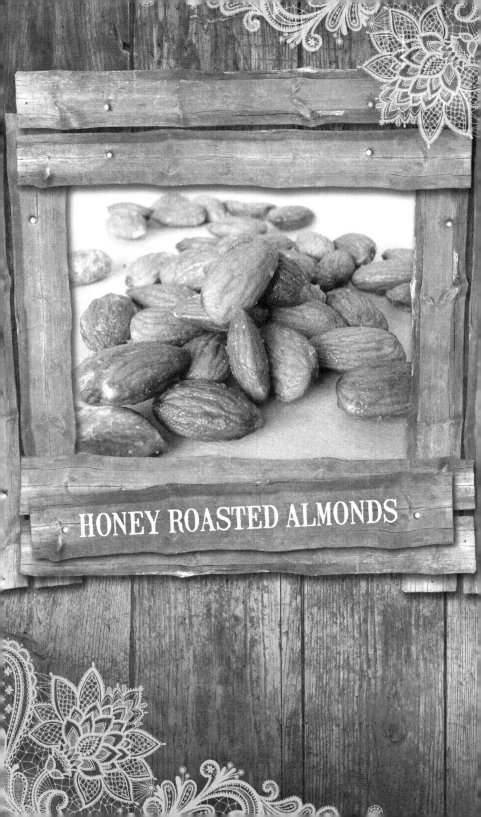

HONEY ROASTED ALMONDS

HONEY ROASTED ALMONDS, OR ROAD FOOD

I keep a bag of these in the center console of my car. Between errands and soccer practice and dance and work and school, kids aren't the only ones who get hungry on the road. This snack is my absolute favorite, and the kids love its salty sweetness.

HONEY ROASTED ALMONDS RECIPE

Ingredients:

- 3 cups raw almonds
- 1 Egg white, whipped
- 2 tbsp raw honey, softened
- 1 tsp avocado oil
- Sea salt to taste

Directions: Preheat oven to 200°F. Place the egg white in the bowl of your stand mixer, and whip until stiff peaks form. Add the honey and oil and whip for a few seconds until blended. Pour in the almonds and turn to coat well.

Spread the coated almonds onto a non-stick rimmed baking sheet and slow roast 4 – 5 hours, turning several times during baking.

Serving Size: ½ cup   Yields: about 6 servings
Prep Time: 10 min   Cook Time: 5 hrs   Total Time: 5 hrs, 10 min

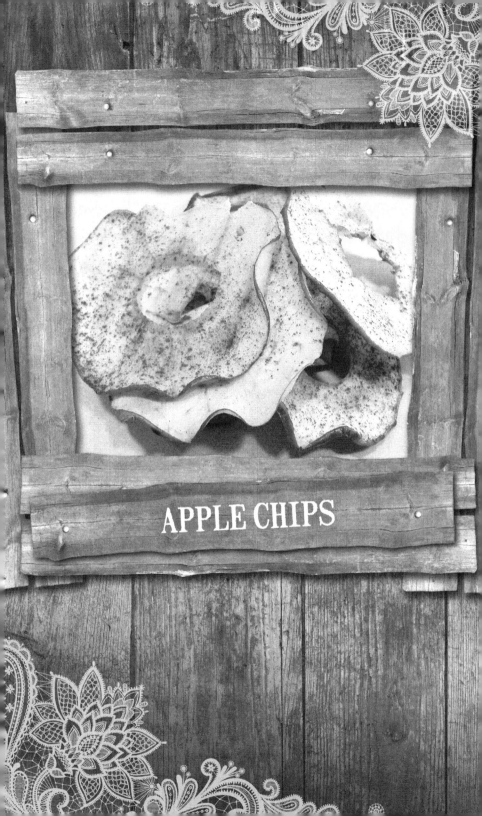

APPLE CHIPS

APPLE CHIPS, OR THE MUNCHIES

Apple chips are so easy to make that I can't bring myself to buy them at the store, not to mention that the prepackaged apple chips almost always contain added sugars and oils. These chips are nothing but apples and cinnamon. For a nice variation, change the cinnamon to chipotle chili powder or pumpkin pie spice!

APPLE CHIPS RECIPE

Ingredients:

- 2 crisp variety apples (Gala, Granny Smith, Golden Delicious, Honey Crisp)
- 1 tsp cinnamon

Directions: Preheat oven to 200°F. Wash and dry the apples. Using a coring tool, remove the core. Slice the apples very thin with a sharp knife or a mandolin.

Lay the apples in a single layer on a wire bakery rack set over a jelly roll pan. Bake for about 2 hours or until the edges are curled and the moisture is removed. Leave on rack to cool, and they will crisp up even more.

Serving Size: 10 chips   Yields: about 3 servings
Prep Time: 5 min   Bake Time: 2 hours
Total Time: 2 hrs 5 min

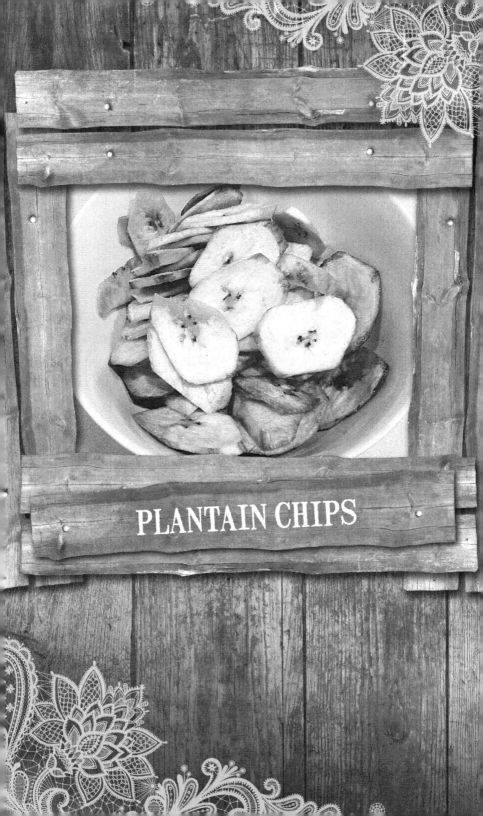

PLANTAIN CHIPS

PLANTAIN CHIPS,
OR SURPRISINGLY GOOD

I wasn't sure about plantains when I first tried them. They looked like big bananas, but not as sweet. When I saw a bag of plantain chips at the health food store, I decided I had to try and make my own Paleo version (cooked in acceptable oil). I bought a bunch, cooked them up, and quickly fell in love with their starchy, crunchy goodness.

For this recipe, it's really important that you use GREEN plantains. If they're too ripe, they will caramelize and you'll end up with a gooey mess.

PLANTAIN CHIP RECIPE

Ingredients:

- 2 large green plantains
- 1 pint coconut oil
- Sea salt to taste

Directions: In a medium heavy saucepan over high heat or a deep fryer, bring the pint of coconut oil to sizzling.

While it's heating, use a paring knife to remove the green peel from the plantain. Slice as thin as possible so your chips stay crunchy.

Drop by the ½ cup batch into the hot oil for 3 – 5 minutes or until sizzling slows and the chips are golden, turning once during cook time. Remove to a plate lined with paper towel to drain. Repeat until all the plantain slices have been cooked.

Season to taste with sea salt or other spices. Allow to cool completely before storing in an airtight container (up to one week).

Serving Size: ¼ cup   Yields: about 6 servings
Prep Time: 5 min   Cook Time: 15 min   Total Time: 20 min

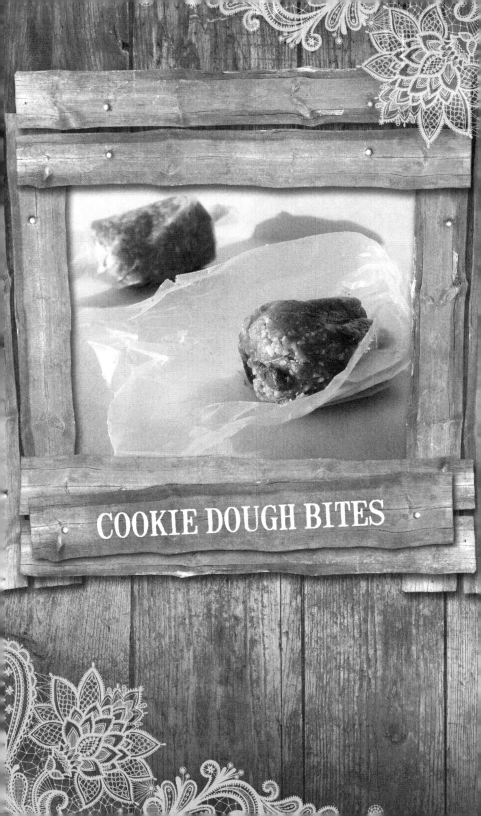

COOKIE DOUGH BITES

COOKIE DOUGH BITES,
OR FIGHT TO THE DEATH

If you're reaching for the last one of these little treats, you'd better watch your back! In our house, we fight to the death (well, not really) over the last tidbit of cookie dough-like goodness. In fact, some of us have been known to stash a few in hiding places for midnight snacking...

I use super-dark chocolate in this recipe, an ingredient that is generally accepted by the Paleo community as a "sometimes treat." However, if you're not doing the dark chocolate, you can easily substitute cacao nibs. They have a chocolate flavor and add crunch to the treat.

Also note that the recipe calls for medjool dates. While you CAN substitute regular dried dates, they're not as sticky so your final product will be a little dryer.

COOKIE DOUGH BITE RECIPE

Ingredients:

- 12 medjool dates, pitted
- 1 cup cashew meal
- 1 tsp vanilla
- 1 oz extra dark chocolate (85% cocoa or higher)

Directions: Place the dates in the food processor and run until they're finely chopped, about a minute. Add the cashew meal and vanilla. Process until a dough lump forms, 2 – 3 minutes. If your dates are too dry (especially if they're not medjool) you can add a bit of water, but not too much.

Add the dark chocolate and pulse a few times to incorporate. Turn the dough onto a piece of waxed paper and press into a rectangle. Cut the dough bites into small squares and wrap each one in waxed paper, twisting on each side like a caramel. Store in a sealed container in the cupboard up to two weeks.

Serving Size: 1 bite   Yields: 12 servings
Prep Time: 10 min   Total Time: 10 min

BREAKFAST TASTIES

ORANGE CRANBERRY SCONES
INSTANT BLUEBERRY HOT BREAKFAST CEREAL
TOASTER PASTRIES

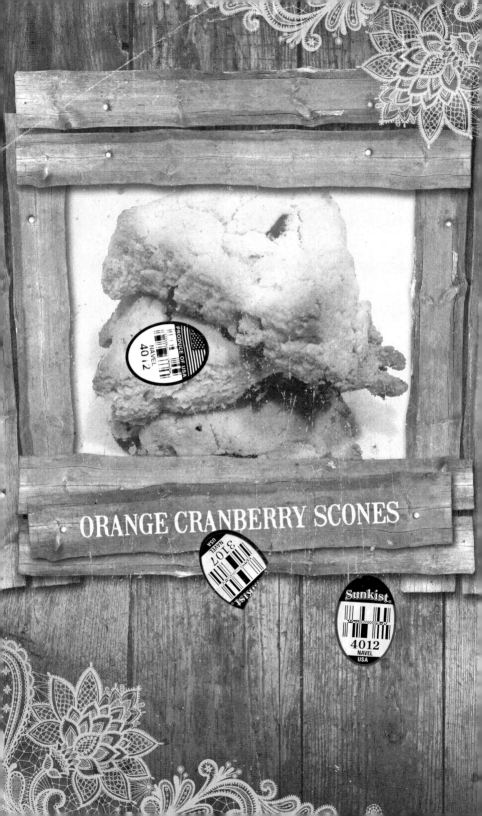

ORANGE CRANBERRY SCONES

ORANGE CRANBERRY SCONES, OR MY QUIET MORNING

I love to wake up before my family, when the house is quiet and the sun has just come up. I sit with a cup of tea and a scone and just prepare myself for the day ahead. These scones are simple to make and stay well in the freezer... just in case you can only catch a quiet morning once in a while.

ORANGE CRANBERRY SCONE RECIPE

Ingredients:

- 2 cups almond flour
- ¼ cup coconut flour
- ¼ cup chopped pecans
- ¼ cup dried cranberries
- 2 tsp baking powder (corn-free, gluten-free)
- 1 Egg
- 2 tbsp fresh orange juice and ½ tsp zest
- 1 tbsp cider vinegar
- 1 tbsp raw honey

Directions: Preheat oven to 350°F. In a medium bowl, mix together the almond flour, coconut flour, and baking powder. Make a well in the center and add the egg, orange juice, zest, cider vinegar, and raw honey. Mix well with a wooden spoon. Mix in the pecans and cranberries.

Turn the dough out onto a piece of parchment paper. Press it into an 8" circle and cut into six wedges, separating them slightly so they're not touching.

Bake for about 16 – 18 minutes until the scones have risen and are golden brown. Cool on a wire rack. Serve warm with whipped grass-fed butter spread and honey or homemade blackberry freezer jam.

Serving Size: 1 scone   Yields: 6 servings
Prep Time: 10 min   Bake Time: 18 min   Total Time: 28 min

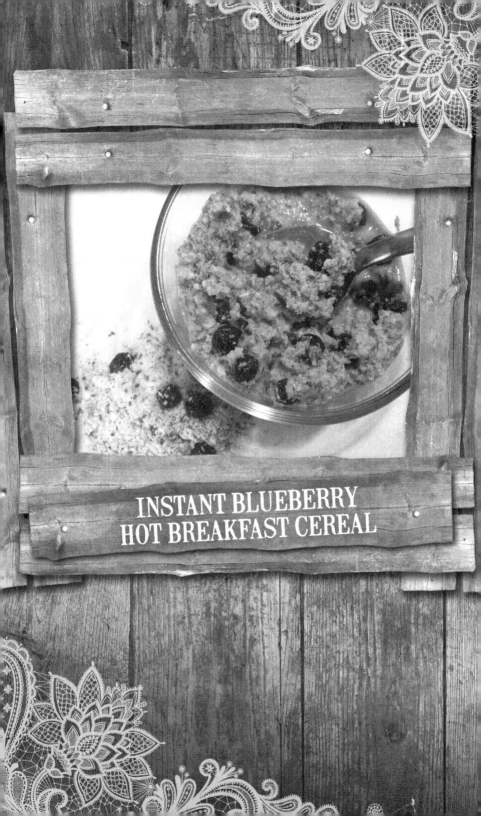

INSTANT BLUEBERRY
HOT BREAKFAST CEREAL

INSTANT BLUEBERRY HOT BREAKFAST CEREAL, OR INDEPENDENCE

There is nothing better than knowing your kids are self-sufficient enough to get up and make their own breakfast... because that means you get to sleep in another hour on Saturday morning! Freeze-dried blueberries work well in this hot "oatmeal-style" cereal, but you could use any freeze-dried or dehydrated fruit.

INSTANT HOT BREAKFAST CEREAL RECIPE

Ingredients:

- 1 cup almond meal
- 1 cup cashew meal
- 1 cup shredded, unsweetened coconut
- 1 cup freeze-dried blueberries
- 4 tsp chia seeds
- 4 tsp birch xylitol, 2 tsp pure stevia, or 4 tsp coconut sugar (optional)
- 1 tsp cinnamon

Directions: Place all ingredients in a large container with a lid and shake to mix well. Store in an airtight container in the cupboard for up to four weeks.

To Prepare: Scoop ½ cup cereal into a bowl. Pour a scant ½ cup boiling water over the cereal. Stir and let sit for about one minute until the liquid is absorbed. Stir and eat!

Serving Size: ½ cup uncooked   Yields: 8 servings
Prep Time: 5 min   Total Time: 5 min

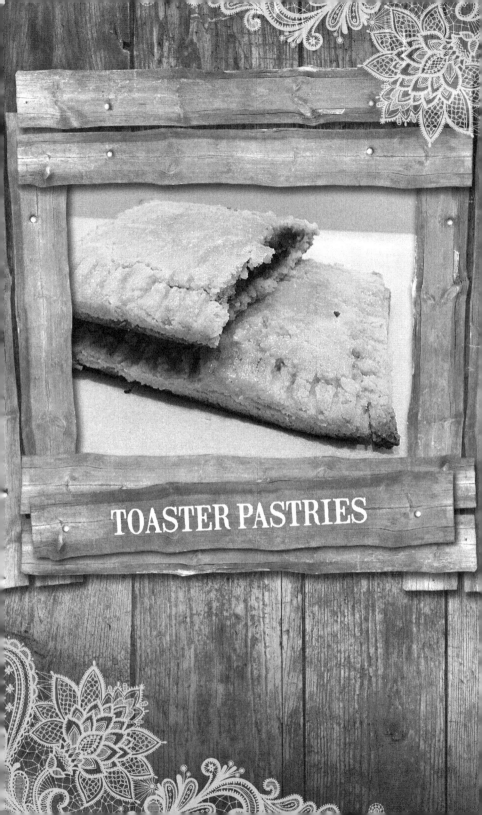

TOASTER PASTRIES

'TOASTER' PASTRIES, OR I STILL LOVE YOU

When you commit your family to the Paleo lifestyle, it's inevitable that you'll end up getting flack somewhere down the road, especially when the kids are older and experiencing the modified food products often consumed in great quantities at birthday parties and school functions. One day, my daughter was begging for pop tarts. She was very upset. When she came home after school that day, she knew how much I loved her... because there sat a plate of these homemade Paleo pop tarts and a tall glass of vanilla almond milk. Everything was well again.

TOASTER PASTRY RECIPE

Ingredients:

- 2 ½ cups blanched almond meal
- ½ cup tapioca starch
- 3 tbsp grass-fed butter
- 1 tbsp raw honey
- 1 egg
- ¼ tsp baking soda
- Egg for egg wash (optional)
- 6 heaping teaspoons apple butter or blackberry jam for filling

Directions: Place the almond meal, tapioca starch, butter, honey, egg and baking soda into the food processor and pulse until a dough-ball forms, about one minute. Turn the dough out onto waxed paper and press into a long, flat rectangle. Wrap in plastic wrap and refrigerate for at least two hours.

Preheat oven to 325°F. On a piece of waxed paper or parchment, roll out the dough and cut eight rectangles of equal size. Place four of them onto a parchment lined baking sheet. Spread each of those four with a teaspoon of filling, leaving a ½" around the edge.

Place a top on each of the filled crusts and press with a fork to seal. Poke a few holes in the top and paint with beaten egg (optional) to give it a golden crust.

Bake for 12 – 15 minutes until the crust is golden brown. Cool on a wire rack. Keep in a paper bag in the cupboard for two days, or refrigerate up to a week.

Serving Size: 1 Pastry   Yields: 4 Servings   Prep Time: 15 min + 2 hours
Bake Time: 15 min   Total Time: 2 ½ hrs

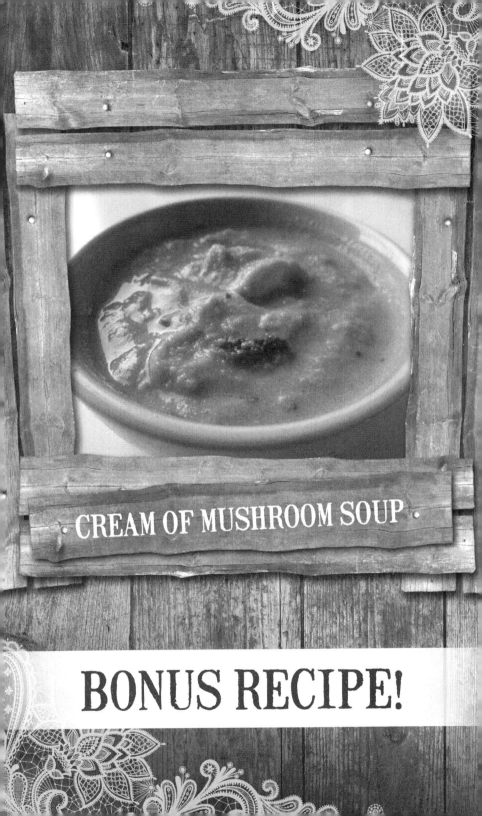

CREAM OF MUSHROOM SOUP

BONUS RECIPE!

CREAM OF MUSHROOM SOUP, OR OH SO CREAMY DREAMY MUSHROOM

This recipe makes cravings for those unhealthy soups in a can a thing of the past. If you love wild mushroom soup, you can easily jazz this up by substituting basic button mushrooms with a mix of Baby Bellas, Oyster mushrooms, Shiitake, Enoki and Cremini, or any combination thereof.

CREAM OF MUSHROOM SOUP RECIPE

Ingredients:

- 1/2 cup sautéed mushrooms (1 cup of fresh mushrooms diced) can use all button mushrooms or make it wild by adding a combination of oyster, shiitake, cremini, enoki and baby bellas
- 1/3 cup dry Paleo soup or sauce mix
- 1 1/4 chicken or beef broth
- 1 tbsp Kerry Gold butter
- Fresh minced garlic (optional)
- Salt and pepper to taste

Directions: First sauté your fresh chopped mushrooms in a sauce pan with 1 tbsp of butter. I also like to add in some fresh minced garlic for some added flavor. After you have sautéed your mushrooms, set aside in a separate bowl.

Next in the same sauce pan mix 1/3 cup dry SOS Save My Sanity Mix with the 1¼ cup of broth in a saucepan on medium heat and whisk together until the sauce is a uniform consistency (no lumps).

Once it is lump free, add your sautéed fresh mushrooms and cook until bubbly. Add salt and pepper to taste. Serve as soup or mix it into your recipe calling for 1 can of cream of mushroom soup.

Freezes well so can be made ahead and frozen for even more convenience.

Serving size 1.5 cups   Yield : 2 servings
Prep Time: 5 min   Cook Time: 5 min   Total Time 10 min

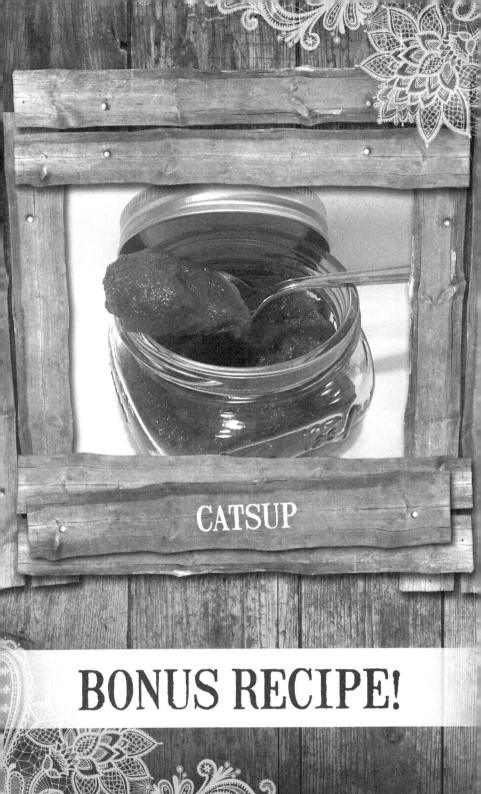

CATSUP

BONUS RECIPE!

PALEO CATSUP
(BONUS RECIPE FROM 'THE PALEO KID')

Catsup isn't just a tasty condiment for French fries and beef. It's also the base for a number of different dips and sauces, like cocktail and BBQ sauces! It's best to make up a big batch of catsup and store it in a jar in the fridge. That way you can dip into it when you need it, rather than having to make it from scratch every time you want to make a sauce that uses it as a base.

PALEO CATSUP RECIPE

Ingredients:

- 10 oz "just prunes" organic baby food
- 10 oz tomato paste
- 3 tsp lemon juice (or unfiltered apple cider vinegar, if using)
- 3 tsp raw honey, softened
- 1/2 tsp ground mustard powder
- 1/2 tsp sea salt

Directions: In a medium sized bowl, whisk all ingredients together until smooth. Store in an airtight container in the refrigerator up to two weeks.

*This is a basic recipe. You can give it your own flare by adding garlic powder, cumin, nutmeg, cinnamon, red chili powder, and more!

Serving size: 1 tbsp   Yields: 20 servings   Prep time: 3 min
Cook time: 0   Total: 3 min

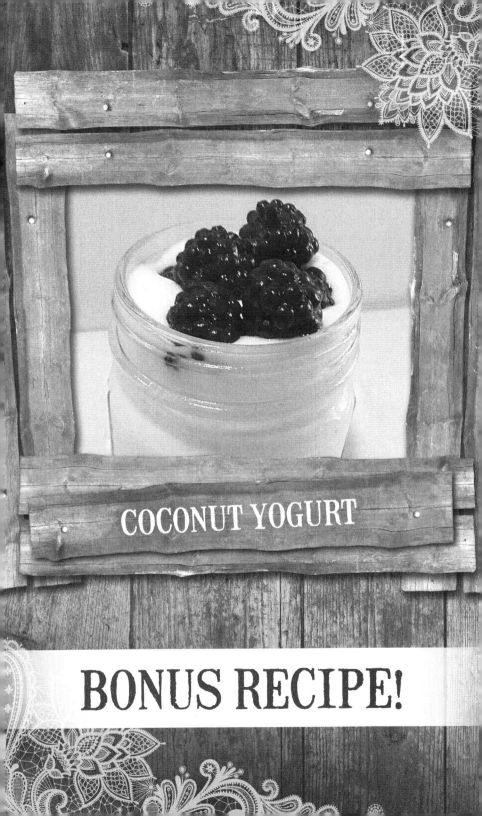

COCONUT YOGURT

BONUS RECIPE!

SLOW COOKER COCONUT YOGURT
(BONUS RECIPE FROM 'PALEO FAST FOOD')

If you're a yogurt fan, this recipe will bring you back to the breakfast table! Coconut milk is the base, and any powdered probiotic provides the bacteria necessary to culture the milk into yogurt. Make sure you don't skip the maple syrup, though. That bacteria needs something to "eat!" I make this each Sunday, because we're usually home and able to easily turn the pot on and off. This way, we start out Monday with a batch of yogurt to last the week! I like to store it in individual cups with fruit on top for breakfast or lunch on the run.

COCONUT YOGURT RECIPE

Ingredients:

- 3 15-0z cans full-fat coconut milk
- 2 tbsp pure maple syrup
- ½ tsp powdered probiotic of choice
- 1 tbsp tapioca starch (optional- for thickening)

Directions: Pour the coconut milk into a slow cooker set on high. Heat for 2 ½ hours, then turn off the slow cooker and allow the milk to come down to room temperature (about 110°F on a candy thermometer). Just walk away and do something else during this time.

Whisk the maple syrup, probiotic of choice, and tapioca starch (if using) into the warm milk. Wrap the entire crock-pot in two layers of thick towel. This helps maintain the temperature. Let it sit overnight. DO NOT open the towels or crock-pot during this time.

In the morning, you have coconut yogurt. If you did not use thickener, the yogurt may be thin. You can thicken it by blending in your favorite fruits in the blender, or by whisking in a little bit of tapioca starch. The yogurt will thicken as it cools.

Pour the yogurt into individual glass jars (topped with fruit, like the blackberries shown here) or into one large airtight container. Store in the refrigerator up to ten days (if you don't gobble it up first).

Serving Size: ½ cup   Yields: 6 servings
Prep Time: 5 min   Slow-Cooker Time: 2 ½ hrs + overnight

ABOUT THE AUTHOR

Kate Evans Scott is the author of the Amazon Bestselling cookbooks The Paleo Kid, Paleo Kid Snacks, The Paleo Kid Lunchbox, The Paleo Kid's Halloween, The Paleo Kid's Christmas and Infused: 26 Spa-Inspired Vitamin Waters.

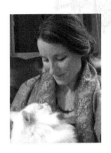

After her son was diagnosed with several food intolerances and after having struggled with her own Autoimmune Disease, Kate made the commitment to remove all grains and processed foods from her family's diet. Her passion and love for good food blossomed after training with a retreat chef in Belgium in her early 20's. Since then, she has wanted to bring her love of food and health into the kitchens of other families struggling with health and dietary challenges.

Kate creates delicious dishes that are suitable for those suffering from digestive and autoimmune diseases - meals that nourish the body while healing the gut. Kate and her husband Mark live in Oregon with their two spirited children.

MORE BY KATE EVANS SCOTT

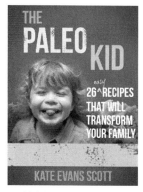

Available Now on Amazon

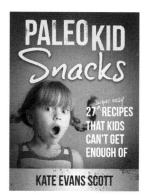

Available Now on Amazon

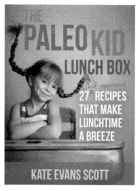

Available Now on Amazon

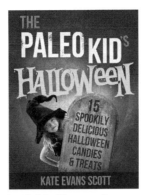

Available Now on Amazon

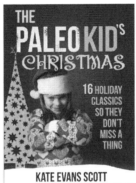

Available Now on Amazon

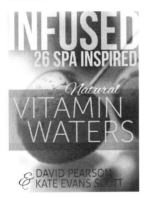

Available Now on Amazon

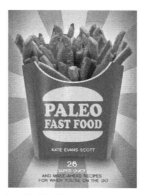

Available Now on Amazon

VISIT:

www.THEPALEOKID.COM

FOR MORE FROM
KIDS LOVE PRESS!

RECIPE NOTES

RECIPE NOTES

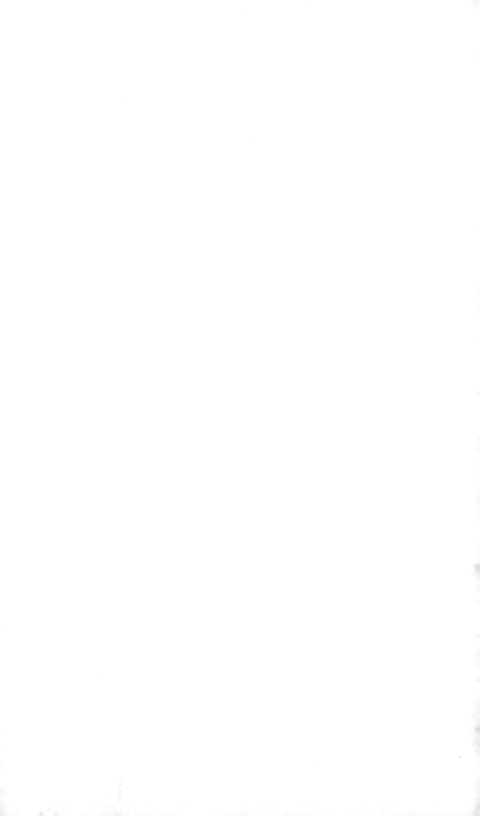

5761941R00050

Printed in Great Britain
by Amazon.co.uk, Ltd.,
Marston Gate.